Asthma and Its prevention.

All you need to know about asthma and its preventions

Ronald M. Kline

Table of Contents

Introduction

Chapter 1: Definition of Asthma

Chapter 2: Causes of Asthma:

Chapter 3: Signs and Symptoms of Asthma

Chapter 4: Types of Asthma

Chapter 5: Control of Asthma

 Conclusion

Introduction

One of the most prevalent chronic inflammatory illnesses is asthma. Its frequency fluctuates between 5 and 20% over the world. Although the exact cause of why some people get asthma and others do not is unknown, it is likely a result of a mix of environmental and hereditary variables. Asthma affects people of all ages and is the most prevalent chronic disease in childhood, adolescence, and adulthood. It has a significant impact on a patient's ability to function well at work and in school. Public health is seriously hampered by asthma. Despite accessible medication, there is no cure, and many individuals are still uncontrolled. To combat this incredibly widespread and spreading illness, interdisciplinary efforts in public health, and fundamental, and clinical research are required.

Chapter 1

Definition of Asthma

Asthma, also known as bronchial asthma, is the most prevalent chronic lung illness in children and is a serious noncommunicable disease (NCD) that affects both children and adults. It is a disorder where a person's airways constrict, swell, and generate excess mucus, all of which make breathing difficult. It is a chronic condition that requires ongoing medical care.

More than 25 million individuals are impacted by it, and it results in roughly 1.6 million trips to the ER. In most situations, it might endure for years or the rest of one's life. It is curable by a licensed medical practitioner, but such a patient requires a medical diagnosis.

Asthma sufferers may encounter the following symptoms:

pressure in the chest

wheezing

breathlessness

coughing

increased production of mucous

Chapter 2

What Causes Asthma?

Although research into the origins of asthma
is ongoing, the following elements are
known to be significant in its development:

family background
The ALA asserts that a person's lifelong risk
of developing asthma may be influenced by
genetics.
A person is more likely than others to get
asthma if one or both of their parents have
the ailment.

Allergies
Particularly if one of their parents has
allergies, some people are more prone to
acquire allergies than others. People who
develop asthma are more likely to have
certain allergic disorders, such as atopic
dermatitis (eczema) or allergic rhinitis (hay
fever).

Respiratory viral infections
Wheezing can be brought on by respiratory issues in childhood and adolescence. Viral respiratory infections in children can lead to the development of persistent asthma.

Workplace exposures
Exposure to specific components at work might aggravate asthma symptoms if you already have them. Additionally, for certain individuals, exposure to specific dust (such as industrial or wood dust), chemical fumes and vapors, and molds might result in the first-ever onset of asthma.

Smoking
Smoking Asthma is most likely to affect smokers. Asthma is also more prevalent in those who were around secondhand smoke or whose moms smoked when they were pregnant. Find out more about how smoking affects asthma sufferers' health.

Air pollution

Exposure to the main component of smog
(ozone) raises the risk for asthma. Urban
dwellers and those who grew up there are
more likely to get asthma.

Obesity
Asthma is more likely to affect fat or
overweight kids and adults. Although the
causes are unknown, some doctors suggest
that being overweight causes low-grade
inflammation in the body. In comparison to
people in a healthy weight range, obese
patients frequently use more drugs,
experience more symptoms, and have
difficulty controlling their asthma.

Chapter 3

Signs and Symptoms of Asthma.

Wheezing is the most typical asthmatic symptom. You may hear a whistling or screeching sound as you breathe.

Other signs of asthma may include:

coughing, particularly at night, when you laugh, or while you're exercising

chest constriction

breathing difficulty

having trouble talking

Panic or anxiety

fatigue

a chest ache

quickly breathing

many infections

difficulty sleeping

Your symptoms may vary depending on the type of asthma you have.

Some folks have symptoms that last all day long. Others might discover that particular hobbies might exacerbate their symptoms.

These specific symptoms are not present in every asthmatic. Make an appointment to visit your doctor if you believe the symptoms you're experiencing might be an indication of an illness like asthma.

Also remember that even with proper management of your asthma, symptoms may still periodically flare up. With the use of quick-acting medications like an inhaler, flare-ups frequently get better, but in more serious situations, they can need medical intervention.

Some indications of an asthma attack include:

coughing

wheezing

voice clearing

inability to sleep

stiffness or discomfort in the chest

weariness.

Chapter 4

Types of Asthma

There are several varieties of asthma, and they include

1. Asthma in children
The most typical chronic disease in kids is asthma. Although it can manifest at any age, children are somewhat more likely to experience it than adults.

The greatest risk for asthma in children in 2019 was between the ages of 12 and 14. 10.8% of people in this age range were affected by the condition. With an average frequency of 9.1%, children aged 5 to 14 had the second-highest prevalence.
In the same year, 8% of those who were 18 years of age or older got asthma.
Some typical causes of pediatric asthma, according to the American Lung Association (ALA), include:

colds and respiratory illnesses
allergies, exposure to cold air, unexpected
temperature changes, excitement, stress,
and exercise. cigarette smoking, especially
secondhand smoke. air pollutants like ozone
and particle pollution.

When a kid enters adulthood, their asthma
may in some situations get better. However,
it is a chronic problem for many people.

2. Asthma in adults
Any age, including maturity, can experience
an asthma attack.

Some elements that can influence an adult's
likelihood of acquiring asthma include

respiratory disease
allergies and contact with allergens
hormonal components
obesity\stress\smoking

3. Work-related asthma

Exposure to an allergen or irritant present at work causes occupational asthma to develop. Working places account for around 1 in 6 adult-onset asthma cases.

About 21% of working persons who have asthma have also noticed that their symptoms became worse at work. An individual may be exposed to asthma triggers in both indoor and outdoor job settings.

4. severe and difficult to manage asthma According to 2014 research, between 5 and 10 percent of asthmatics suffer severe asthma.

For causes unrelated to asthma, some people experience severe symptoms. For instance, kids might not yet know how to use an inhaler properly.

Others suffer from persistent, severe asthma. In certain situations, treating asthma with large doses of medicine or using inhalers properly does not work. 3.6% of persons who have asthma may have this kind of asthma.

Another kind of asthma, eosinophilic asthma, may not respond to standard treatments in severe instances. Others with eosinophilic asthma may benefit from particular biologic therapy, even if others control their condition with conventional asthma drugs.

A particular biologic drug lowers the number of eosinophils, a kind of blood cell implicated in an allergic response that can cause asthma.

5. Seasonal asthma
In reaction to allergens that are only present in the environment during specific seasons of the year, this form of asthma develops.

Seasonal asthma symptoms, for instance, may be exacerbated by chilly winter air or spring or summer pollen.

Those who have seasonal asthma continue to have it throughout the rest of the year, although they often do not exhibit symptoms.

Chapter 5

Control of Asthma

You must take all reasonable steps to reduce your exposure to asthma triggers if you have asthma. To do this, you must first understand what makes you cough, wheeze, and struggle for breath. There is no known treatment for asthma, but there are things you can do to manage it and avoid attacks.

1. Recognize asthma triggers

An asthmatic symptom cascade can be triggered by specific asthma triggers. These consist of:

allergens in the air
icy air
the flu or cold virus
Exercise\sSinusitis
Smoke\sFragrances

Finding your asthma triggers and taking preventative measures to avoid them is essential.

For many weeks, record your symptoms in an asthma diary. List all the physical and psychological factors that have an impact on your asthma. Examine the journal after an asthma episode to see what, if anything, may have contributed to it. Molds and cockroaches are two typical asthma causes that aren't usually visible. Get more information about allergy testing from your asthma expert. Take action to avoid them after that.

Take precautions to avoid an asthma attack if you have exercise-induced asthma, are preparing for a strenuous workout, or want to exercise in cold, humid, or dry conditions. To treat your asthma, heed the instructions of your doctor (usually by using an asthma inhaler containing the drug albuterol before you exercise).

2. Steer clear of allergens

It's crucial to avoid allergens (items you're allergic to) if you suffer from allergies and asthma. Exposure to allergens might temporarily worsen the inflammation in your airways, increasing the likelihood of an attack.

3. Avoid All Forms of Smoke

Asthma and smoke don't mix well. Reduce your exposure to any smoke, including that from cigarettes, incense, candles, fires, and fireworks. Avoid going to public locations where smoking is permitted and don't allow it in your house or automobile. If you smoke, seek assistance to stop. Asthma is usually worse by smoking.

4. Avoid colds

Try your best to stay healthy. Stay away from persons who are contagious since doing so will make your asthma symptoms worse. If you handle anything that a person with a respiratory infection may have touched, thoroughly wash your hands.

5. Home Allergy-Proofing

There are steps you can do to make your surroundings allergy-proof and reduce your risk of an asthma attack, whether you're at home, at work, or on the road. Avoid eating at establishments that allow or are smokey. Book a non-smoking hotel room. If at all possible, bring your bedding and pillows in case the hotel only has down comforters and feather pillows available. They can aggravate asthma symptoms and harbor dust mites.

6. Vaccinate yourself.

To protect yourself against the flu virus, which can make your asthma worse for days or weeks, get a flu vaccination every year. You are more likely to require hospitalization for the flu and its complications, such as pneumonia if you have asthma. Every five to ten years, adults over 19 should have the Pneumovax vaccination against pneumonia. Additionally, you are more likely to get pneumococcal pneumonia, common bacterial pneumonia. You also require a Tdap vaccination to shield you from tetanus, diphtheria, and whooping cough, as well as a zoster vaccination, to shield you from shingles.

7. Use asthma medications exactly as directed. Long-term asthma treatments are intended to stop attacks and symptoms. Even if you are symptom-free, you must take them daily. They'll reduce airway inflammation and keep your asthma under control, making flare-ups less probable. Talk to your doctor about switching to a different treatment if side effects annoy you.

8. Adherence to Your Asthma Action Plan Even if you feel OK, take your medications. Maintain a portable inhaler. Check your plan for advice on what drugs to take if you start to have symptoms.

The strategy can advise you on the best medications to take during an attack and when to contact your doctor.

Conclusion

In conclusion, asthma may be characterized as a chronic respiratory disorder that manifests as chest tightness, wheezing, trouble breathing, and coughing. The main episodes required to diagnose asthma diagnosis are tightening and swelling of the airways as well as an increase in mucus production. Asthma is also diagnosed by physical examinations, lung function testing, blood tests, and chest X-rays. Symptom preventers and symptom controllers are the drugs used to manage asthma long-term. Medication for symptom relief is used to treat the condition's symptoms right away. To prevent and lessen asthma episodes, healthcare practitioners must educate their patients about the risk factors for asthma, which include occupational variables like dust and chemicals, cold weather exposure, exercise, infections, and inhalation or ingestion of allergens and pollutants. The physical, psychological, and social welfare of the client is impacted by chronic asthma disorders.

www.ingramcontent.com/pod-product-compliance
Lightning Source LLC
Chambersburg PA
CBHW051728250726

48653CB00008B/3262